Unique Dash Diet for Beginners:

Full Guide on Dash Diet, How It Works; Dash Meal Plan for a Week; What to Consume; Dos & Don'ts, Plus Some Salient Questions You Would What to Ask & Lots More

By

Doctor Peter L. Turnbull

Copyright@2020

TABLE OF CONTENTS

CHAPTER ONE

INTRODUCTION

Meaning of DASH Diet:

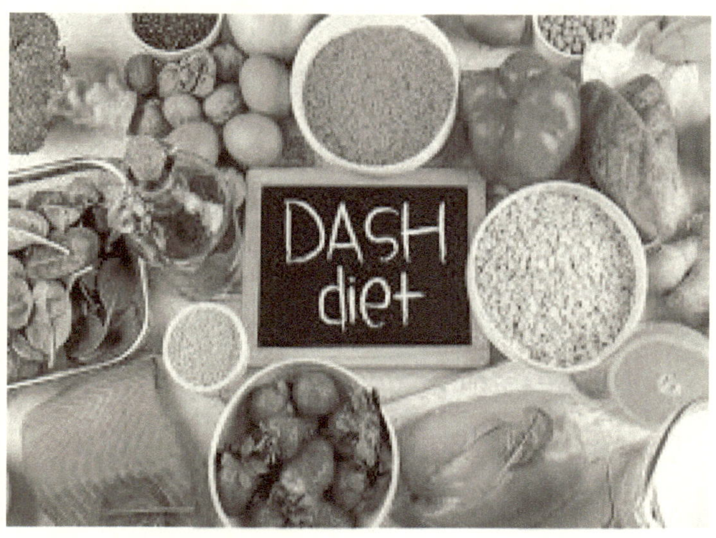

DASH represents Dietary Approaches to Stop Hypertension. It is an eating plan that depends on research contemplates supported by the National Heart, Lung, and Blood Institute (NHLBI). These investigations demonstrated that DASH brings down hypertension and improves levels of cholesterol. This lessens your danger of getting coronary illness.

The DASH eating plan:

•   Emphasizes vegetables, organic products, and entire grains

•   Includes sans fat or low-fat dairy items, fish, poultry, beans, nuts, and vegetable oils

- Limits nourishments that are high in soaked fat. These nourishments incorporate greasy meats, full-fat dairy items, and tropical oils, for example, coconut, palm part, and palm oils.

- Limits sugar-improved drinks and desserts

Alongside DASH, other way of life changes can help bring down your circulatory strain. They incorporate remaining at a sound weight, working out, and not smoking.

The DASH diet is particularly suggested for individuals with (hypertension) or prehypertension.

The DASH diet eating plan has been demonstrated to bring down circulatory strain in considers supported by the National Institutes of Health (Dietary Approaches to Stop Hypertension). Notwithstanding being a low salt (or low sodium) plan, the DASH diet gives extra advantages to diminish circulatory strain. It depends on an eating plan wealthy in foods grown from the ground, and low-fat or non-fat dairy, with entire grains. It is a high fiber, low to direct fat eating regimen, rich in potassium, calcium, and magnesium. The full DASH diet plan is appeared here. The DASH diet is a solid arrangement, intended for the entire family. New examination keeps on demonstrating extra medical advantages of the arrangement.

Notwithstanding being suggested by your doctor, DASH is additionally embraced by:

- The US Nationwide Heart, Lung, As well as Blood Institute

- The American Heart Association (AHA)

- The 2015 Dietary Guidelines for Americans

- US rules for treatment of hypertension

- Treatment Guidelines for Women regarding 2011 AHA

- The Mayo Clinic

- The DASH eating plan has been demonstrated to bring down pulse in only 14 days, even without bringing down sodium consumption. Best reaction came in individuals whose circulatory strain was just decently high, incorporating those with prehypertension. For individuals with progressively serious hypertension, who will most likely be unable to dispose of medicine, the DASH diet can help improve reaction to prescription, and assist lower with blooding pressure. The DASH diet can help lower cholesterol, and with weight reduction and exercise, can decrease insulin obstruction and lessen the danger of creating diabetes.

More Explanation on DASH Diet

Dietary Approaches to Stop Hypertension, or DASH, is an eating regimen prescribed for individuals who need to forestall or treat hypertension — otherwise called hypertension — and lessen their danger of coronary illness.

The DASH diet centers around organic products, vegetables, entire grains and lean meats.

The eating regimen was made after scientists saw that hypertension was considerably less basic in individuals who followed a plant-based eating routine, for example, veggie lovers and vegans

That is the reason the DASH diet underscores products of the soil while containing some lean protein sources like chicken, fish and beans. The eating routine is low in red meat, salt, included sugars and fat.

Researchers accept that one of the principle reasons individuals with hypertension can profit by this eating regimen is on the grounds that it diminishes salt admission.

The ordinary DASH diet program energizes close to 1 teaspoon (2,300 mg) of sodium every day, which is in accordance with most national rules.

The lower-salt adaptation suggests close to 3/4 teaspoon (1,500 mg) of sodium every day.

Summary for You

The DASH diet was intended to lessen hypertension. While wealthy in organic products, vegetables and lean proteins, it limits red meat, salt, included sugars and fat.

CHAPTER TWO

BENEFITS OF DASH DIET

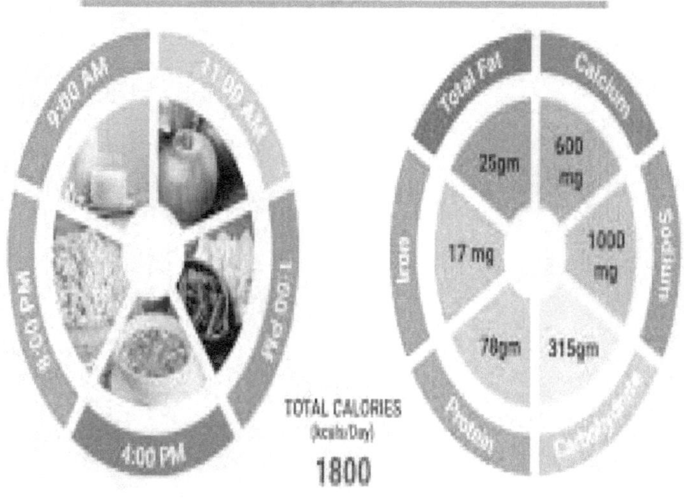

Past lessening circulatory strain, the DASH diet offers various possible advantages, including weight reduction and decreased disease chance.

Be that as it may, you shouldn't anticipate that DASH should assist you with shedding weight all alone —

as it was structured in a general sense to bring down circulatory strain. Weight reduction may just be an additional advantage.

The eating routine effects your body in a few different ways.

Brings Down Blood Pressure

Circulatory strain is a proportion of the power put on your veins and organs as your blood goes through them. It's included in two numbers:

- Systolic pressure: The weight in your veins when your heart thumps.

- Diastolic pressure: The weight in your veins between pulses, when your heart is very still.

Typical circulatory strain for grown-ups is a systolic weight under 120 mmHg and a diastolic weight under 80 mmHg. This is regularly composed with the systolic circulatory strain over the diastolic weight, this way: 120/80.

Individuals with a circulatory strain perusing of 140/90 are considered to have hypertension.

Strangely, the DASH diet obviously brings down circulatory strain in both sound individuals and those with hypertension.

In contemplates, individuals on the DASH diet despite everything experienced lower circulatory strain regardless of whether they didn't shed pounds or limit salt admission However, when sodium admission was confined, the DASH diet brought down pulse much further. Actually, the best decreases in pulse were

found in individuals with the most
minimal salt utilization

These low-salt DASH diet results were
generally noteworthy in individuals
who previously had hypertension,
diminishing systolic circulatory strain
by a normal of 12 mmHg and diastolic
pulse by 5 mmHg

In individuals with ordinary pulse, it
diminished systolic circulatory strain
by 4 mmHg and diastolic by 2 mmHg

This is in accordance with different investigations which uncover that confining salt admission can decrease circulatory strain — particularly in the individuals who have hypertension

Remember that an abatement in circulatory strain doesn't generally mean a diminished danger of coronary illness

May Aid Weight Loss
You will probably encounter lower circulatory strain on the DASH diet whether you get thinner.

Be that as it may, in the event that
you as of now have hypertension,
odds are you have been encouraged to
get in shape.

This is on the grounds that the more
you gauge, the higher your pulse is
probably going to be.

Also, getting in shape has been
appeared to bring down circulatory
strain.

A few investigations recommend that individuals can get in shape on the DASH diet. However, the individuals who have shed pounds on the DASH diet have been in a controlled calorie shortfall — which means they were advised to eat less calories than they were exhausting.

Given that the DASH diet removes a great deal of high-fat, sweet nourishments, individuals may find that they consequently decrease their calorie very demands and get thinner. Others may need to deliberately confine their admission.

In any case, in the event that you need to get more fit on the DASH diet, you'll despite everything need to go on a calorie-decreased eating regimen.

Other Potential /Great Health Benefits

DASH diet/meal may likewise influence different zones of wellbeing. The eating regimen:

•	Decreases malignant growth hazard: An ongoing survey showed that individuals following the DASH diet had a lower danger of certain tumors, including colorectal and bosom disease

•	Lowers metabolic condition hazard: Some investigations note that the DASH diet lessens your danger of metabolic disorder by up to 81%

•	Lowers diabetes chance: The eating routine has been connected to a lower danger of type 2 diabetes. A

few investigations show that it can
improve insulin obstruction too

•	Decreases coronary illness
hazard: In one late audit in ladies,
following a DASH-like eating regimen
was related with a 20% lower danger
of coronary illness and a 29% lower
danger of stroke

A considerable lot of these defensive
impacts are credited to the eating
regimen's high leafy foods content.
When all is said in done, eating more

foods grown from the ground can
help lessen danger of malady

Summary for You

DASH brings down circulatory strain
— especially in the event that you
have raised levels — and may help
with weight reduction. It could
decrease your danger of diabetes,
coronary illness, metabolic disorder
and a few tumors.

CHAPTER THREE

THE WORKING PRINCILES OF DASH DIET, WHAT TO CONSUME AND LOTS MORE

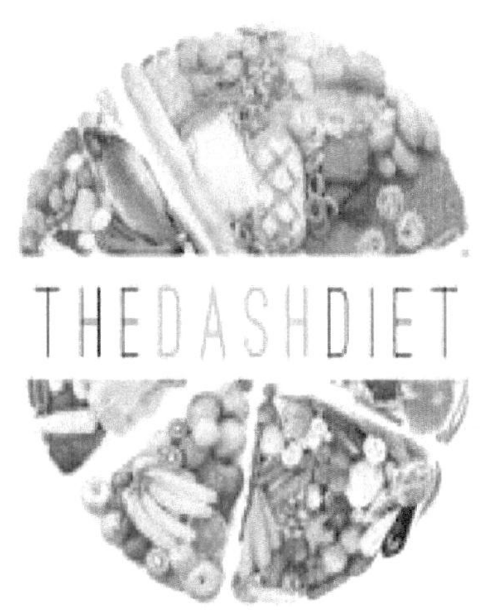

Accomplishes It Work for Everyone?

While concentrates on the DASH diet established that the best decreases in circulatory strain happened in those with the most reduced salt admission, the advantages of salt limitation on wellbeing and life expectancy are not satisfactory cut.

For individuals with hypertension, diminishing salt admission altogether influences circulatory strain. In any case, in individuals with ordinary circulatory strain, the impacts of diminishing salt admission are a lot littler.

The hypothesis that a few people are salt delicate — implying that salt applies a more noteworthy impact on their circulatory strain — could incompletely clarify this.

Summary for You

If your salt admission is high, bringing it down gives significant medical advantages. Far reaching salt limitation, as exhorted on the DASH diet, may just be useful for individuals who are salt touchy or have hypertension.

Confining Salt Too Much Is Not Good for You

Eating too minimal salt has been connected to medical issues, for example, an expanded danger of coronary illness, insulin obstruction and liquid maintenance.

The low-salt form of the DASH diet suggests that individuals eat close to 3/4 teaspoon (1,500 mg) of sodium every day.

Nonetheless, it's hazy whether there are any advantages to decreasing salt admission this low — even in individuals with hypertension

Truth be told, an ongoing survey found no connection between salt admission and danger of death from

coronary illness, in spite of the way
that bringing down salt admission
caused an unobtrusive decrease in
circulatory strain.

Be that as it may, in light of the fact
that a great many people eat a lot of
salt, bringing down your salt
admission from extremely high
measures of 2–2.5 teaspoons (10–12
grams) a day to 1–1.25 teaspoons (5–6
grams) a day might be helpful.

This objective can be accomplished
effectively by decreasing the measure
of profoundly handled food in your
eating regimen and eating for the
most part the entire nourishments.

Summary for You

Although decreasing salt admission from handled nourishments is gainful for a great many people, eating too minimal salt may likewise be unsafe.

What to Eat on the Diet

The DASH diet doesn't list explicit nourishments to eat. Rather, it suggests explicit servings of various nutritional categories.

The quantity of servings you can eat relies upon what number of calories you expend. The following is a case of food divides dependent on a 2,000-calorie diet.

Entire Grains: 6–8 Servings for each Day

Instances of entire grains incorporate entire wheat or entire grain breads, entire grain breakfast oats, earthy colored rice, bulgur, quinoa and oats.

Instances of a serving include:

•   1 cut of entire grain bread

•   1 ounce (28 grams) of dry, entire grain oat

•   1/2 cup (95 grams) of cooked rice, pasta or grain

Vegetables: 4–5 Servings for each Day

All vegetables are permitted on the DASH diet.

Instances of a serving include:

•   1 cup (around 30 grams) of crude, verdant green vegetables like spinach or kale

•   1/2 cup (around 45 grams) of cut vegetables — crude or cooked — like broccoli, carrots, squash or tomatoes

Natural products: 4–5 Servings for each Day

In case you're following the DASH approach, you'll be eating a ton of natural product. Instances of organic products you can eat incorporate apples, pears, peaches, berries and tropical natural products like pineapple and mango.

Instances of a serving include:

*   1 medium apple

*   1/4 cup (50 grams) of dried apricots

•   1/2 cup (30 grams) of new, solidified or canned peaches

Dairy Products: 2–3 Servings for every Day

Dairy items on the DASH diet ought to be low in fat. Models incorporate skim milk and low-fat cheddar and yogurt.

Instances of a serving include:

•   One cup of fat milk that is low in fat(240 ml)

- One cup of fat yogurt that is low in fat, (285 grams)

- 1.5 ounces (45 grams) of low-fat cheddar

Lean Chicken, Meat and Fish: 6 or Fewer Servings for each Day

Pick lean slices of meat and attempt to eat a serving of red meat just every so often — close to a few times per week.

Instances of a serving include:

- 1 ounce (28 grams) of cooked meat, chicken or fish

- 1 egg

Nuts, Seeds and Legumes: 4-5 Servings for each Week

These incorporate almonds, peanuts, hazelnuts, pecans, sunflower seeds, flaxseeds, kidney beans, lentils and split peas.

Instances of a serving include:

- 1/3 cup (50 grams) of nuts

•   2 tablespoons (40 grams) of nut spread

•   2 tablespoons (16 grams) of seeds

•   1/2 cup (40 grams) of cooked vegetables

Fats and Oils: 2–3 Servings for each Day

The DASH diet suggests vegetable oils over different oils. These incorporate margarines and oils like canola, corn, olive or safflower. It additionally suggests low-fat mayonnaise and light serving of mixed greens dressing.

Instances of a serving include:

•   1 teaspoon (4.5 grams) of delicate margarine

•   1 teaspoon (5 ml) of vegetable oil

•   1 tablespoon (15 grams) of mayonnaise

•   2 tablespoons (30 ml) of plate of mixed greens dressing

Candy and Added Sugars: 5 or Fewer Servings for each Week

Added sugars are kept to a base on the DASH diet, so limit your admission of treats, pop and table sugar. The DASH diet additionally limits grungy sugars and elective sugar sources, similar to agave nectar.

Instances of a serving include:

- 1 tablespoon (12.5 grams) of sugar

- 1 tablespoon (20 grams) of jam or jam

- 1 cup (240 ml) of lemonade

Summary for You

The DASH diet doesn't list explicit nourishments to eat. Rather, it's a dietary example concentrated on servings of nutrition types.

CHAPTER FOUR

A WHOLE WEEK EXAMPLE OF DASH DIET FOR YOU

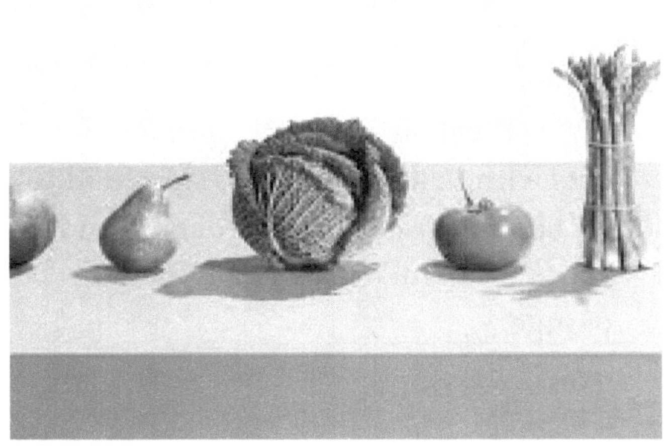

Test Menu for One Week

Here's a case of a one-week feast plan — in light of 2,000 calories for every day — for the normal DASH diet:

Monday

•	Breakfast: 1 cup (90 grams) of oats with 1 cup (240 ml) of skim milk, 1/2 cup (75 grams) of blueberries and 1/2 cup (120 ml) of new squeezed orange.

•	Snack: An apple that is not too big as well as one of cup of fat yogurt that is low in fat (285 grams)

- Lunch: Tuna and mayonnaise sandwich made with 2 cuts of entire grain bread, 1 tablespoon (15 grams) of mayonnaise, 1.5 cups (113 grams) of green plate of mixed greens and 3 ounces (80 grams) of canned fish.

- Snack: 1 medium banana.

- Dinner: 3 ounces (85 grams) of lean chicken bosom cooked in 1 teaspoon (5 ml) of vegetable oil with 1/2 cup (75 grams) every one of broccoli and carrots. Presented with 1 cup (190 grams) of earthy colored rice.

Tuesday

- Breakfast: 2 cuts of entire wheat toast with 1 teaspoon (4.5 grams) of margarine, 1 tablespoon (20 grams) of jam or jam, 1/2 cup (120 ml) of new squeezed orange and 1 medium apple.

- Snack: 1 medium banana.

- Lunch: 3 ounces (85 grams) of lean chicken bosom with 2 cups (150 grams) of green plate of mixed greens, 1.5 ounces (45 grams) of low-fat cheddar and 1 cup (190 grams) of earthy colored rice.

- Snack: 1/2 cup (30 grams) of canned peaches and 1 cup (285 grams) of low-fat yogurt.

•	Dinner: 3 ounces (85 grams) of salmon cooked in 1 teaspoon (5 ml) of vegetable oil with 1 cup (300 grams) of bubbled potatoes and 1.5 cups (225 grams) of bubbled vegetables.

Wednesday

•	Breakfast: 1 cup (90 grams) of oats with 1 cup (240 ml) of skim milk and 1/2 cup (75 grams) of blueberries. 1/2 cup (120 ml) of new squeezed orange.

•	Snack: 1 medium orange.

•	Lunch: 2 cuts of entire wheat bread, 3 ounces (85 grams) of lean turkey, 1.5 ounces (45 grams) of low-fat cheddar, 1/2 cup (38 grams) of green plate of mixed greens and 1/2 cup (38 grams) of cherry tomatoes.

•	Snack: 4 entire grain wafers with 1.5 ounces (45 grams) of curds and 1/2 cup (75 grams) of canned pineapple.

•	Dinner: 6 ounces (170 grams) of cod filet, 1 cup (200 grams) of pureed potatoes, 1/2 cup (75 grams) of green peas and 1/2 cup (75 grams) of broccoli.

Thursday

•   Breakfast: 1 cup (90 grams) of oats with 1 cup (240 ml) of skim milk and 1/2 cup (75 grams) of raspberries. 1/2 cup (120 ml) of new squeezed orange.

•   Snack: 1 medium banana.

•   Lunch: Salad made with 4.5 ounces (130 grams) of flame broiled fish, 1 bubbled egg, 2 cups (152 grams) of green serving of mixed greens, 1/2 cup of cherry tomatoes, (38 grams) as well as two tablespoons of fat dressing that is low in fat, (30 ml).

•   Snack: 1/2 cup (30 grams) of canned pears and 1 cup (285 grams) of low-fat yogurt.

•	Dinner: 3 ounces (85 grams) of pork filet with 1 cup (150 grams) of blended vegetables and 1 cup (190 grams) of earthy colored rice.

Friday

•	Breakfast: 2 bubbled eggs, 2 cuts of turkey bacon with 1/2 cup (38 grams) of cherry tomatoes, 1/2 cup (80 grams) of heated beans and 2 cuts of entire wheat toast, in addition to 1/2 cup (120 ml) of new squeezed orange.

•	Snack: 1 medium apple.

- Lunch: 2 cuts of entire wheat toast, 1 tablespoon of low-fat mayonnaise, 1.5 ounces (45 grams) of low-fat cheddar, 1/2 cup (38 grams) of serving of mixed greens and 1/2 cup of cherry tomatoes, (38 grams).

- Snack: 1 cup of organic product serving of mixed greens.

- Dinner: Spaghetti plus meatballs created with one cup of spaghetti, (190 grams) as well as minced turkey, 4 ounces (115 grams). 1/2 cup of green peas, (75 grams) which is an afterthought.

Saturday

- Breakfast: 2 cuts of entire wheat toast with 2 tablespoons (40 grams) of nutty spread, 1 medium banana, 2 tablespoons (16 grams) of blended seeds and 1/2 cup (120 ml) of new squeezed orange.

- Snack: 1 medium apple.

- Lunch: 3 ounces (85 grams) of flame broiled chicken, 1 cup (150 grams) of cooked vegetables and 1 cup (190 grams) couscous.

- Snack: 1/2 cup (30 grams) of blended berries and 1 cup (285 grams) of low-fat yogurt.

- Dinner: 3 ounces (85 grams) of pork steak and 1 cup (150 grams) of ratatouille with 1 cup (190 grams) of earthy colored rice, 1/2 cup (40 grams) of lentils and 1.5 ounces (45 grams) of low-fat cheddar.

- Dessert: Low-fat chocolate pudding.

Sunday

- Breakfast: 1 cup (90 grams) of oats with 1 cup (240 ml) of skim milk, 1/2 cup (75 grams) of blueberries and 1/2 cup (120 ml) of new squeezed orange.

- Snack: 1 medium pear.

- Lunch: Chicken plate of mixed greens made with 3 ounces (85 grams) of lean chicken bosom, 1 tablespoon of mayonnaise, 2 cups (150 grams) of green serving of mixed greens, 1/2 cup (75 grams) of cherry tomatoes, 1/2 tablespoon (4 grams) of seeds and 4 entire grain saltines.

- Snack: 1 banana and 1/2 cup (70 grams) of almonds.

- Dinner: 3 ounces of dish meat with 1 cup (150 grams) of bubbled potatoes, 1/2 cup (75 grams) of broccoli and 1/2 cup (75 grams) of green peas.

Summary for You

On the DASH diet, you can eat an
assortment of luscious, solid dinners
that pack a lot of vegetables nearby
different foods grown from the
ground protein sources.

CHAPTER FIVE

ALLOWING ONE'S DIET/MEAL TO BE MORE OF DASH STUFF PLUS SOME QUESTIONS YOU WOULD LIKE TO ASK

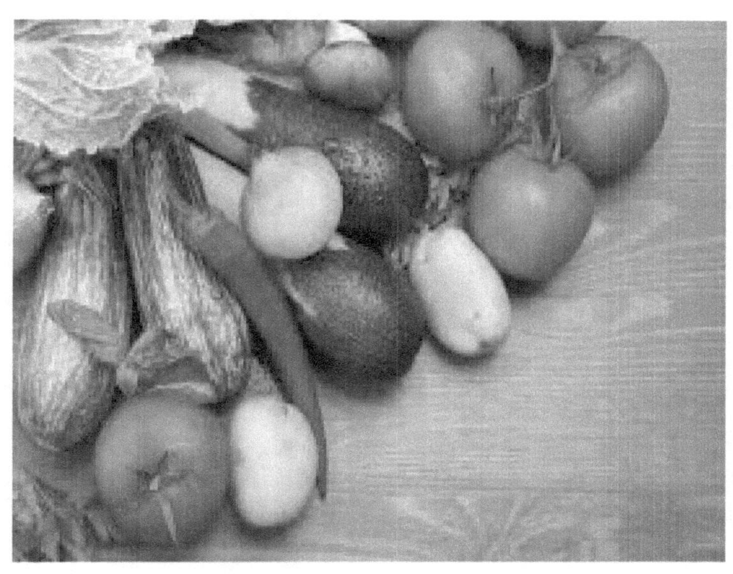

Guidelines to Create Your Diet That is More of DASH-Meal Related

Since there are no set nourishments on the DASH diet, you can adjust your present eating routine to the DASH rules by doing the accompanying:

• Eat more vegetables and organic products.

•	Swap refined grains for entire grains.

•	Choose sans fat or low-fat dairy items.

•	Pick from protein(lean) sources such as fish, beans, and poultry.

•	Cook with vegetable oils.

- Limit your admission of nourishments high in included sugars, similar to pop and candy.

- Limit your admission of nourishments high in immersed fats like greasy meats, full-fat dairy and oils like coconut and palm oil.

Outside of estimated new organic product juice parcels, this eating regimen prescribes you stick to low-calorie drinks like water, tea and espresso.

Summary for You

It's conceivable to adjust your present eating routine to the DASH diet. Just eat more leafy foods, pick low-fat items just as lean proteins and breaking point your admission of handled, high-fat and sweet nourishments.

Often Asked Questions

In case you're contemplating attempting DASH to bring down your circulatory strain, you may have a couple of inquiries concerning different parts of your way of life.

The most usually posed inquiries are tended to beneath.

Would I be able to Drink Coffee on the DASH Diet?

The DASH diet doesn't endorse explicit rules for espresso. In any case, a few people stress that energized refreshments like espresso may build their circulatory strain.

It's notable that caffeine can cause a transient increment in circulatory strain

Besides, this ascent is more prominent in individuals with hypertension

Be that as it may, an ongoing survey guaranteed that this well-known drink doesn't expand the drawn out danger of hypertension or coronary illness — despite the fact that it caused a present moment (1–3 hours) increment in circulatory strain

For most sound individuals with typical circulatory strain, 3–4 customary cups of espresso every day are viewed as protected

Remember that the slight ascent in pulse (5–10 mm Hg) brought about by caffeine implies that individuals who as of now have hypertension most likely should be increasingly cautious with their espresso utilization.

Do I Require to Exercise Right on the DASH Meal or Diet?

The DASH diet is considerably powerful at bringing down circulatory strain when matched with physical movement.

Given the autonomous advantages of activity on wellbeing, this isn't unexpected.

It's prescribed to complete 30 minutes of moderate action most days, and it's essential to pick something you appreciate — along these lines, you will be bound to keep it up.

Instances of moderate movement
include:

•   Brisk strolling (15 minutes for
every mile or 9 minutes for every
kilometer)

•   Running (10 minutes for every
mile or 6 minutes for each kilometer)

•   Cycling (6 minutes for every
mile or 4 minutes for each kilometer)

- Swimming laps (20 minutes)

- Housework (an hour)

Would i be able to Drink Alcohol on the DASH Diet?

Drinking an excess of liquor can expand your circulatory strain

Indeed, consistently drinking multiple beverages every day has been connected to an expanded danger of hypertension and coronary illness

On the DASH diet, you should drink liquor sparingly and not surpass official rules — 2 or less beverages for each day for men and 1 or less for ladies.

Summary for You

You can drink espresso and liquor with some restraint on the DASH diet. Joining the DASH diet with exercise may make it considerably or increasingly powerful.

CHAPTER SIX

DASH MEAL PLAN FOR YOUR WELL-BEING

WHAT CAN YOU EAT?

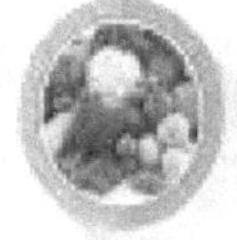

VEGETABLES

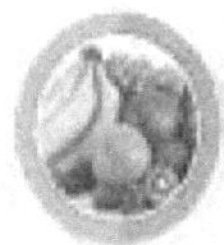

FRUIT

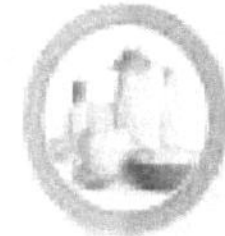

LOW FAT DAIRY

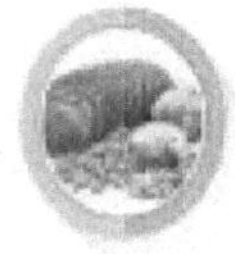

WHOLE GRAINS

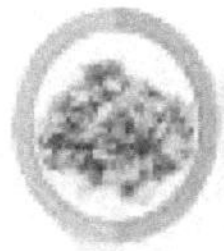

SEEDS, NUTS & LEGUMES

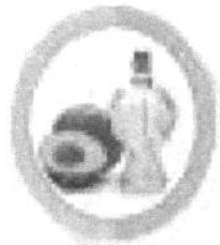

FATS & OILS

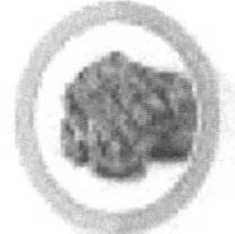

LEAN MEAT, FISH & POULTRY.

Guidelines to follow a DASH Diet Plan:

The DASH diet plan center around expanding vegetables, natural products, entire grains, and vegetables; picking lean meats, low-fat dairy, nuts and solid fats; and restricting included sugars, trans fats, included salt, and prepared nourishments. Serving sizes from every nutrition class depend on singular calorie needs (see beneath for a 1600-calorie plan), and you'll likely find that the arrangement looks quite near the My Plate plan, just as another reliably appraised "top eating regimen," the Mediterranean Diet. Here's a breakdown of the suggested supplements in a common day and week on the DASH diet:

Supplements per Day:

- Grains: 6 servings

- Vegetables: 3-4 servings

- Fruits: 4 servings

- Low-Fat or Fat-Free Dairy: 2-3 servings

- Meat(lean) plus Poultry, or Fish: Four ounces or perhaps less

- Fat/oils: 2 servings

- Sodium: 2300 mg or less

Supplements per Week:

•	Nuts, seeds, and vegetables: 3-4 times each week

•	Sweets and included sugars: 3 servings or less

The key to DASH's prosperity is its accentuation on expanding vegetables, organic products, and entire nourishments that are normally low in sodium and high in potassium. While most realize that diminishing sodium is fundamental, many don't understand that getting satisfactory potassium admission is similarly as key for directing circulatory strain.

At the point when nourishments are prepared, their potassium levels really decline. In this way, picking entire or insignificantly prepared nourishments can improve circulatory strain guideline from both a sodium and a potassium point of view. What's more, you'll as a rule decline your admission of soaked fat, included sugars, and generally speaking calories—all of which can assist you with getting in shape, and keep it off for good.

CHAPTER SEVEN
CONCLUSION

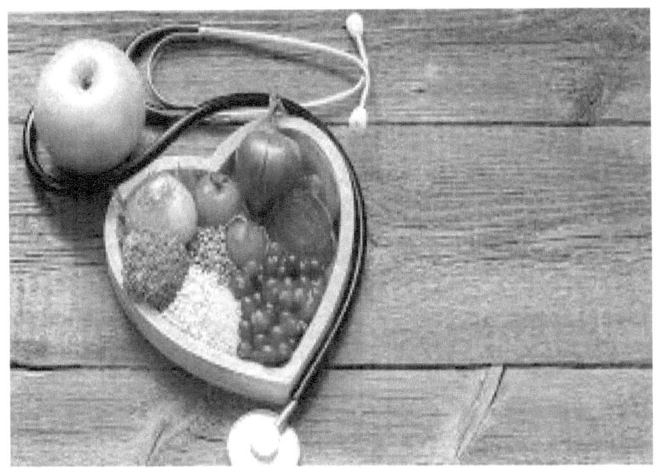

The DASH diet might be a simple and viable approach to diminish circulatory strain.

Be that as it may, remember that slicing every day salt admission to 3/4 teaspoon (1,500 mg) or less has not been connected to any hard medical advantages —, for example, a diminished danger of coronary illness — regardless of the way that it can bring down circulatory strain.

Additionally, the DASH diet is fundamentally the same as the standard low-fat eating routine, which huge controlled preliminaries have not appeared to lessen the danger of death by coronary illness

Sound people may have little motivation to follow this eating routine. In any case, on the off chance that you have hypertension or figure you might be delicate to salt, DASH might be a decent decision for you.

Happy DASH Diet eating!

THE END